Improving Focus with Natural Supplements:

Lion's Mane, Fo-Ti, Pine Bark, Turmeric, Saffron, Magnesium, Vitamin D, and B Complex and more.

Jeannine M. Petrilak

Skyblupink

Table of Contents:

1. Combining Forces For Overall Brain Health

Combining a variety of natural supplements can be a holistic approach to enhancing focus, cognitive function, and overall brain health. Here's an updated guide on how to safely combine supplements, including the addition of new ingredients, and a sample daily regimen for optimal focus.

Safe Combination of Supplements for Enhanced Focus:
When combining supplements, it's crucial to consider their individual benefits, potential synergies, and any possible interactions. Here's an overview of the supplements and their roles:

B-Complex Vitamins: B vitamins are essential for energy production, neurotransmitter synthesis, and overall brain function. They work synergistically to support cognitive health.

Magnesium: Magnesium is a key mineral for cognitive function, mood regulation, and relaxation. It enhances the effects of B vitamins and supports nerve function.

Vitamin D: Vitamin D plays a vital role in cognitive health, mood, and energy levels. It works in harmony with B vitamins and magnesium to optimize brain function.

Lion's Mane (Hericium erinaceus): Lion's Mane is a powerful medicinal mushroom known for its neuroprotective and cognitive-enhancing properties. It can improve focus, memory, and overall brain health.

Pine Bark (Pycnogenol): Pine Bark extract is rich in antioxidants and improves blood flow to the brain, enhancing cognitive function and reducing mental fatigue.

Cat's Claw (Uncaria tomentosa): Cat's Claw is a traditional herb with potential cognitive benefits. It may support focus, memory, and overall brain health.

Saffron: Saffron is a spice with neuroprotective properties. It has been shown to improve mood, enhance cognitive function, and reduce symptoms of depression and anxiety.

Panax Ginseng: Panax Ginseng is an adaptogenic herb known for its ability to enhance mental performance, improve focus, and reduce mental fatigue.

Shilajit: Shilajit is a natural substance rich in fulvic acid and minerals. It has been used traditionally to enhance cognitive function, improve energy levels, and support overall brain health.

Omega-3 Fatty Acids: Omega-3s, in the form of 1 tablespoon of chia seeds soaked in water, provide essential fatty acids that are crucial for brain health. They support cognitive function, reduce inflammation, and improve focus.

Garlic: Garlic is a powerful herb with antioxidant and anti-inflammatory properties. It may help improve cognitive function and protect against cognitive decline.

Chlorella: Chlorella is a type of freshwater algae that is rich in nutrients. It has been shown to have cognitive-enhancing properties and may improve focus and mental clarity.

Synergies and Interactions:

The combination of these supplements creates a powerful synergy, enhancing their individual benefits and creating a holistic approach to cognitive health. For instance:

B vitamins, magnesium, and Vitamin D work together to support energy production, neurotransmitter synthesis, and cognitive function.

Lion's Mane and Pine Bark can enhance each other's neuroprotective effects, improving focus and memory.

Cat's Claw and Shilajit may complement each other, providing additional cognitive support and potential anti-inflammatory benefits.

Saffron and Panax Ginseng can work synergistically to improve mood, reduce anxiety, and enhance cognitive performance.

Omega-3 fatty acids from chia seeds provide essential nutrients for brain health, supporting the function of all other supplements.

Sample Daily Supplement Regimen for Focus Enhancement:

Here's a suggested daily supplement regimen to enhance focus and cognitive function:

B-Complex Vitamins: Take a high-quality B-complex supplement containing the full spectrum of B vitamins, preferably in their methylated forms.

Magnesium: Opt for a highly absorbable form like magnesium glycinate or magnesium L-threonate. Take 200-400 mg daily with food.

Vitamin D: Choose a Vitamin D3 supplement. The dosage can vary, but a general guideline is 1000-2000 IU daily. Consult a healthcare professional for personalized advice.

Lion's Mane: Take a Lion's Mane supplement containing at least 500 mg of the mushroom extract.

Pine Bark: Opt for a Pine Bark extract with a standardized dosage of at least 100 mg.

Cat's Claw: Choose a Cat's Claw supplement with a standardized dosage of at least 500 mg.

Saffron: Add a pinch of saffron to your daily diet or take a saffron extract supplement as directed.

Panax Ginseng: Take a Panax Ginseng supplement as directed, typically 1-2 grams daily.

Shilajit: Opt for a high-quality Shilajit supplement, following the recommended dosage.

Omega-3 Fatty Acids: Soak 1 tablespoon of chia seeds in water overnight. Consume the chia gel, which provides a good source of Omega-3s.

Garlic: Include garlic in your daily diet or take a garlic supplement as directed.

Chlorella: Take a Chlorella supplement as directed, typically 1-2 grams daily.

Importance of Cycling Supplements and Detoxification:

Cycling supplements and incorporating detoxification practices can be beneficial for several reasons:

Cycling supplements: Taking breaks from certain supplements allows the body to adjust and prevents potential tolerance. It also gives the body a chance to reset and optimize its natural processes.

Detoxification: As suggested by Dr. Klinghardt, detoxification can be an essential aspect of improving focus and cognitive function. Detoxification practices, such as intermittent fasting, saunas, and herbal support, can help eliminate toxins and support overall brain health.

Individualization: Everyone's needs are unique, so it's important to adjust the dosages and supplement combinations based on individual responses and health status.

Professional guidance: Consulting a healthcare professional, especially one with expertise in natural medicine, can provide personalized advice and ensure the safety and efficacy of your supplement regimen.

In conclusion, this holistic approach to enhancing focus combines a variety of natural supplements, each with its unique benefits. By understanding the synergies and interactions between these supplements, and with the guidance of a healthcare professional, individuals can create a personalized regimen to support their cognitive health and overall well-being.

2. Importance of Focus and Cognitive Health

Focus and cognitive health are fundamental to productivity, creativity, and overall quality of life. When we're able to concentrate, it's easier to learn, problem-solve, make decisions, and retain information—all of which are essential skills in personal and professional settings. Cognitive health, which encompasses memory, reasoning, and executive functions, allows us to navigate complex situations, handle stress effectively, and stay engaged with our tasks.

Maintaining a sharp mind becomes even more crucial as we age. With age, natural cognitive decline can lead to decreased memory, slower processing speed, and challenges in sustaining attention. By supporting focus and cognitive health early on, we can potentially stave off age-related cognitive issues, maintain mental agility, and continue to perform at our best. A healthy mind is also key to emotional well-being, as focus and cognitive resilience play a role in managing stress, anxiety, and mood.

Modern Challenges to Maintaining Focus

In our fast-paced, technology-driven world, maintaining focus has become increasingly challenging. Many aspects of modern life contribute to these challenges:

- **Digital Overload**: The constant notifications, emails, and messages from devices can quickly become overwhelming. Research shows that frequent interruptions disrupt focus, reduce productivity, and make it difficult to return to deep, uninterrupted work.
- **Information Overload**: The internet provides access to endless amounts of information, which, while beneficial, can lead to mental fatigue. Constantly processing large amounts of information can make it difficult to discern

what's important, leading to scattered focus and reduced memory retention.

- **Chronic Stress**: Many individuals face high levels of stress from work, relationships, and societal expectations. Chronic stress increases cortisol, which can impair memory, reduce focus, and even lead to brain fog and exhaustion.
- **Sleep Deprivation**: Busy schedules and the demands of daily life can lead to sleep loss, and sleep deprivation has a profound impact on cognitive function. Lack of sleep impairs attention, memory consolidation, and decision-making.
- **Poor Nutrition and Sedentary Lifestyle**: A diet low in essential nutrients and a sedentary lifestyle can negatively affect the brain's ability to stay alert and focused. The brain requires certain vitamins, minerals, and healthy fats to function optimally, and regular physical activity has been shown to improve mental clarity and focus.

Role of Natural Supplements in Enhancing Focus

Given these challenges, many people are turning to natural supplements as a safe and holistic way to support focus and cognitive health. Natural supplements like Lion's Mane, Fo-Ti, Pine Bark, and essential vitamins and minerals are gaining popularity for their potential to improve attention, memory, and overall mental resilience. Recommended for further reading: Finally Focused by Dr. James Greenblatt.

Natural supplements often contain compounds that work synergistically with the body's own processes to support brain health:

- **Supporting Brain Function and Neuroplasticity**: Supplements like Lion's Mane and Pine Bark contain compounds that may promote neuroplasticity, or the brain's ability to form and reorganize connections. This can lead to better memory retention and improved cognitive flexibility.

- **Reducing Inflammation and Oxidative Stress**: Chronic inflammation and oxidative stress are detrimental to cognitive health. Supplements like Turmeric (with its active compound, curcumin) and Pine Bark Extract are known for their anti-inflammatory and antioxidant properties, which can help protect brain cells from damage and support long-term cognitive health.

- **Enhancing Energy Production and Neurotransmitter Function**: Vitamins such as B Complex and minerals like magnesium play essential roles in cellular energy production and neurotransmitter synthesis. These nutrients can improve mental clarity and reduce brain fog by supporting efficient brain signaling and energy metabolism.

- **Regulating Mood and Stress Levels**: Chronic stress and mood fluctuations can severely impact focus. Adaptogenic herbs like Fo-Ti help the body adapt to stress, reducing cortisol levels and promoting a calmer, more focused mind. Vitamin D also plays a role in mood regulation and has been linked to cognitive function, especially in areas related to attention and mental resilience.

Incorporating these natural supplements, alongside lifestyle improvements, can make a significant difference in cognitive health and focus. However, they are most effective when combined with healthy habits like regular exercise, a balanced diet, quality sleep, and mindful time management. Consulting a healthcare provider before starting any supplement regimen is also crucial to ensure these choices are safe and personalized for individual needs.

3. Lion's Mane Mushroom

Overview and Origins

Lion's Mane Mushroom (*Hericium erinaceus*) is a unique, white, shaggy mushroom resembling the mane of a lion, which is how it got its distinctive name. Traditionally used in Asian medicine, Lion's Mane has been highly valued in China, Japan, and Korea for centuries, where it's known as *Yamabushitake* in Japan and *Hou Tou Gu* in China. This mushroom grows naturally on hardwood trees in temperate forests and has long been prized not only as a culinary ingredient but also for its medicinal properties. In recent years, scientific interest has focused on its potential cognitive benefits, particularly its effects on memory, focus, and mental clarity.

Benefits for Cognitive Function and Nerve Growth

Lion's Mane is rich in bioactive compounds that support brain health, most notably hericenones and erinacines. These compounds have been found to stimulate the production of nerve growth factor (NGF), a protein essential for the growth, maintenance, and survival of neurons. NGF is crucial for neurogenesis—the brain's ability to create new neurons and neural connections—which plays a key role in memory, learning, and overall cognitive function.

Some of the primary benefits of Lion's Mane for cognitive health include:

- **Enhanced Memory and Learning**: Lion's Mane has been shown to support memory formation and retention, likely due to its effects on neurogenesis.
- **Improved Focus and Mental Clarity**: By supporting NGF production and reducing oxidative stress, Lion's

Mane may enhance focus and reduce brain fog, leading to clearer thinking and faster processing.

- **Mood Regulation and Neuroprotection**: Some studies suggest that Lion's Mane may have antidepressant and anti-anxiety effects, potentially linked to its ability to support neuroplasticity and reduce inflammation in the brain. This can also help people stay more relaxed, which indirectly improves focus.

Research on Lion's Mane and Its Impact on Focus and Memory

Studies show Lion's Mane has promising effects on cognitive health:

- **Cognitive Function in Older Adults**: A 2009 Japanese study found that adults aged 50-80 with mild cognitive impairment experienced improved cognitive function after 16 weeks of Lion's Mane supplementation. However, these benefits declined once the supplement was stopped, suggesting that ongoing use may be necessary for sustained effects.

- **Neurogenesis in Animals**: Animal studies suggest that Lion's Mane may stimulate neurogenesis, especially in the hippocampus (a region tied to memory and learning), potentially enhancing memory and learning with regular use.

- **Mood and Anxiety Reduction**: In a 2010 study, menopausal women who consumed Lion's Mane reported reduced anxiety and depression after 4 weeks. Since reduced anxiety can improve focus, this mood-boosting effect may indirectly support mental clarity and sustained attention.

Suggested Dosages and Forms

Lion's Mane is available in various forms, including capsules, powders, and teas, making it easy to incorporate into daily routines. Here's a look at the common forms and suggested dosages:

- **Capsules**: Capsules are convenient and widely available. A typical daily dosage ranges from 500 mg to 3,000 mg, depending on the concentration. It's advisable to start at the lower end and gradually increase as needed.
- **Powders**: Many people add Lion's Mane powder to smoothies, coffee, or other beverages. The dosage usually ranges from 1-3 grams per day. Some powders are double-extracted (water and alcohol), which can provide a broader spectrum of Lion's Mane's bioactive compounds.
- **Teas and Tinctures**: Lion's Mane tea is another way to consume this mushroom, though dosage control can be less precise. Tinctures, often alcohol-based, offer a concentrated form that can be added to water or taken directly. Follow the manufacturer's recommendations.

For cognitive benefits, Lion's Mane should be taken consistently. Some users report noticeable improvements within weeks, while for others, it may take several months of consistent use.

Possible Side Effects and Considerations

Lion's Mane is generally considered safe, with minimal reported side effects. However, it's essential to consider the following:

- **Digestive Upset**: Some individuals may experience mild digestive discomfort, including nausea or stomach cramps, especially when first starting Lion's Mane or if taking high doses. Starting with a low dose and gradually increasing can help reduce this risk.

- **Allergic Reactions**: Although rare, there have been reports of allergic reactions to Lion's Mane, particularly among people with mushroom allergies. Symptoms may include skin rash, itching, or respiratory issues. If you have a history of mushroom allergies, consult a healthcare provider before using Lion's Mane.
- **Interactions with Medication**: Lion's Mane may interact with certain medications, particularly those that affect the immune system. As it can have mild immune-modulating effects, it's wise to check with a healthcare professional if you're on immunosuppressants or other related medications.

In summary, Lion's Mane is a promising natural supplement for cognitive enhancement, backed by traditional use and emerging scientific research. By promoting nerve growth and reducing brain inflammation, it has the potential to improve memory, focus, and mental clarity.

4. Fo-Ti (He Shou Wu)

Background and Traditional Uses in Chinese Medicine

Fo-Ti, also known as *He Shou Wu* or *Polygonum multiflorum*, is a popular herb in traditional Chinese medicine, revered for its supposed anti-aging and longevity-promoting effects. Its name, *He Shou Wu*, translates to "Mr. He's Black Hair," referencing the legend of an older man whose hair turned black again after regularly consuming this herb. Traditionally, Fo-Ti has been used to nourish the kidneys and liver, strengthen the body, improve vitality, and promote mental clarity.

Adaptogenic Properties and How It Supports Focus

As an adaptogen, Fo-Ti helps the body manage stress by balancing cortisol levels and supporting the adrenal glands, making it easier to stay focused and mentally resilient under pressure. This balancing effect on the stress response can prevent mental fatigue, improve focus, and enhance endurance, especially during demanding tasks. Adaptogens like Fo-Ti work by modulating the body's stress response, which helps create a stable environment for cognitive processes.

Antioxidant Effects and Neuroprotective Benefits

Fo-Ti is rich in antioxidants, particularly compounds such as resveratrol and flavonoids, which help protect brain cells from oxidative stress and inflammation. These antioxidants combat free radicals, which can damage neurons and accelerate cognitive decline. By protecting against oxidative damage, Fo-Ti may slow down age-related brain changes, thus supporting long-term cognitive health.

Additionally, Fo-Ti has shown neuroprotective properties by supporting mitochondrial health (the powerhouses of cells), which is vital for energy production and overall brain vitality. This neuroprotection may also support memory and mental clarity.

Evidence on Cognitive Enhancement

While human studies on Fo-Ti's direct effects on cognition are limited, some animal research suggests that it may enhance learning, memory, and overall cognitive function. For example, studies on aged rats have demonstrated improved memory performance following Fo-Ti supplementation, along with reduced oxidative stress markers in the brain. Though more research on humans is needed, these findings indicate potential cognitive benefits, especially with long-term use.

Recommended Dosages and Formulations

Fo-Ti is commonly available in several forms, including raw root powder, processed (cured) root, capsules, and tinctures. Processed Fo-Ti (cured with black beans) is generally preferred, as it is considered less harsh on the liver and more suitable for long-term use.

- **Dosage**: Typical dosages range from 500 mg to 1,500 mg per day, depending on the formulation and individual health goals. Always follow product instructions, as potency can vary.
- **Formulations**: Capsules and tinctures are convenient and standardized, while raw powders can be mixed into beverages. It's often advised to start with a lower dose and gradually increase as needed.

Precautions and Interactions

While Fo-Ti is generally considered safe, there are a few precautions to keep in mind:

- **Liver Health**: Rare cases of liver toxicity have been reported, primarily with high doses of unprocessed Fo-Ti.

Choosing processed (cured) Fo-Ti and using it within recommended dosages can help mitigate this risk.

- **Medication Interactions**: Fo-Ti may interact with medications metabolized by the liver or those affecting liver enzymes. If you're taking medications, particularly for liver conditions, consult a healthcare provider before starting Fo-Ti.
- **Pregnancy and Nursing**: Fo-Ti is not recommended for pregnant or breastfeeding women due to insufficient safety data.

In summary, Fo-Ti is a traditional herb with adaptogenic, antioxidant, and neuroprotective benefits that can potentially support focus, stress resilience, and overall cognitive health. However, as with any supplement, it's wise to start with a conservative dose and consult a healthcare provider, especially if there are pre-existing conditions or medications involved.

5. Pine Bark Extract (Pycnogenol)

What is Pycnogenol? History and Extraction Process

Pycnogenol is a natural plant extract derived from the bark of the French maritime pine tree (*Pinus pinaster*), which grows along the coast of southwest France. Used for centuries in traditional medicine, Pycnogenol is now widely recognized for its potent antioxidant and anti-inflammatory properties. The extract is standardized to contain a high concentration of procyanidins, bioflavonoids, and organic acids, which contribute to its wide range of health benefits.

The extraction process involves careful harvesting of the bark and using a water-based extraction method, ensuring that the extract is free from solvents or additives. This high-quality extraction yields a concentrated form of Pycnogenol that retains its natural antioxidant compounds, making it ideal for supplementation.

The Science Behind Its Antioxidant Power

Pycnogenol is one of the most powerful natural antioxidants available, boasting a complex combination of procyanidins, bioflavonoids, and phenolic acids. These compounds neutralize free radicals, which are harmful molecules that can damage cells and accelerate aging. By reducing oxidative stress, Pycnogenol protects brain cells from damage, which can enhance cognitive function over time. The antioxidant power of Pycnogenol is considered particularly beneficial for reducing inflammation, which is increasingly linked to cognitive decline and neurodegenerative diseases.

Effects on Blood Flow and Brain Function

One of Pycnogenol's unique benefits is its ability to improve blood flow, particularly by enhancing endothelial function (the function of blood vessel linings). It stimulates the production of nitric oxide, a molecule that relaxes blood vessels and improves circulation. Better blood flow means more oxygen and nutrients are delivered to the brain, which can support mental clarity, focus, and overall brain function.

By enhancing circulation, Pycnogenol also aids in reducing symptoms of cognitive fatigue and mental fog, promoting clearer thinking and sustained attention, especially during demanding tasks.

Studies Linking Pine Bark to Improved Attention and Focus

Several studies have explored Pycnogenol's benefits for cognitive performance, particularly in areas related to attention and memory:

- **ADHD and Attention**: A 2006 study on children with ADHD found that those taking Pycnogenol showed significant improvements in attention, visual-motor coordination, and concentration compared to a placebo group. These improvements were linked to Pycnogenol's antioxidant effects and its ability to enhance blood flow to the brain.

- **Memory and Cognitive Performance in Adults**: In a 2012 study, older adults taking Pycnogenol for three months showed improvements in memory, attention, and executive function compared to a placebo group. Researchers noted that the extract's effects on blood flow likely contributed to these cognitive benefits.

- **Reducing Test Anxiety and Improving Focus in Students**: A 2008 study on college students found that those who supplemented with Pycnogenol experienced reduced test anxiety and improved test performance. The study highlighted Pycnogenol's role in stabilizing stress levels, which can contribute to better focus and mental resilience under pressure.

These findings suggest that Pycnogenol can support various aspects of cognitive performance, including memory, attention, and mental stamina.

How to Take Pine Bark for Cognitive Support

Pycnogenol is typically available in capsule or tablet form, making it convenient for daily use. For cognitive support, doses usually range between **50 mg and 200 mg per day**. Here are some guidelines:

- **Start Small**: Begin with a lower dose, such as 50 mg per day, and gradually increase if needed, monitoring how it affects your focus and energy levels.
- **Timing**: Pycnogenol can be taken with or without food. Some people prefer taking it in the morning to support mental clarity and focus throughout the day.

It's often recommended to take Pycnogenol consistently for at least 4-6 weeks to notice cognitive effects, as its benefits can build up over time.

Safety, Side Effects, and Contraindications

Pycnogenol is generally considered safe when taken within recommended dosages. However, some people may experience mild side effects, including:

- **Digestive Upset**: Mild gastrointestinal symptoms such as nausea, stomach discomfort, or diarrhea may occur, particularly at higher doses.
- **Headaches and Dizziness**: Rarely, some individuals report headaches or mild dizziness.

Pycnogenol may interact with certain medications, particularly blood thinners and antiplatelet drugs, as it can have mild blood-thinning effects. Additionally, those with autoimmune conditions or on immunosuppressive drugs should exercise caution, as Pycnogenol can modulate the immune response.

In summary, Pycnogenol is a powerful natural supplement with antioxidant, anti-inflammatory, and blood flow-enhancing properties that can support focus, memory, and mental clarity. It's generally safe for long-term use but should be used carefully in those with certain medical conditions or who are on specific medications. Always consult a healthcare provider before beginning Pycnogenol supplementation, especially if you're on medication or have underlying health concerns.

6. Turmeric and Curcumin

Background: Curcumin as the Active Compound in Turmeric

Turmeric, a bright yellow-orange spice commonly used in Indian cuisine, is derived from the root of the *Curcuma longa* plant. It has been used for thousands of years in Ayurvedic and traditional medicine for its medicinal properties. The primary active compound in turmeric, curcumin, is responsible for many of its health benefits. Curcumin is a potent antioxidant and anti-inflammatory agent, known for its positive effects on the brain and body. However, curcumin only makes up a small percentage of turmeric by weight (about 3-5%), which is why concentrated curcumin extracts are often used for therapeutic purposes.

How Curcumin Supports Brain Health and Reduces Inflammation

Curcumin has powerful anti-inflammatory effects that protect brain health. Chronic inflammation has been linked to cognitive decline, mood disorders, and neurodegenerative diseases like Alzheimer's. Curcumin inhibits inflammatory pathways and reduces the production of pro-inflammatory molecules in the brain, helping to prevent damage to brain cells and preserve cognitive function.

In addition, curcumin has strong antioxidant properties, neutralizing free radicals that can cause oxidative stress in the brain. By reducing both inflammation and oxidative stress, curcumin helps maintain a healthy environment for neurons and supports neurogenesis (the growth of new neurons), which is critical for memory, learning, and overall mental clarity.

Impact on Mental Clarity and Focus, Backed by Research

Research has shown that curcumin can have a positive effect on cognitive function, especially in areas related to memory, mood, and mental clarity:

- **Cognitive Function in Older Adults**: In a 2018 study conducted at UCLA, participants aged 50-90 who took curcumin twice daily for 18 months showed significant improvements in memory and attention compared to a placebo group. MRI scans revealed fewer signs of brain degeneration in those taking curcumin, suggesting its neuroprotective potential.

- **Mood and Reduced Anxiety**: A study published in 2015 found that curcumin supplementation helped reduce symptoms of depression and anxiety in people with major depressive disorder. Because mood and focus are often interconnected, improved mood can lead to clearer thinking and enhanced mental resilience.

- **Improved Blood Flow**: Curcumin has also been shown to improve blood flow, including to the brain. Enhanced blood flow ensures that the brain receives more oxygen and nutrients, which can support mental clarity, reduce fatigue, and improve focus.

These findings underscore curcumin's ability to support cognitive function, especially in older adults, and highlight its potential benefits for both focus and mental clarity.

Best Ways to Take Turmeric for Brain Benefits (with Black Pepper and Fats for Better Absorption)

Curcumin on its own has poor bioavailability, meaning that it's not easily absorbed by the body. However, there are ways to significantly enhance its absorption:

- **Combine with Black Pepper**: Black pepper contains piperine, a compound that can increase curcumin absorption by up to 2,000%. Many high-quality curcumin supplements include piperine for this reason.

- **Take with Healthy Fats**: Curcumin is fat-soluble, so consuming it with healthy fats, like those found in coconut oil, olive oil, or avocado, can improve its absorption.

- **Choose Enhanced Formulations**: Some curcumin supplements use advanced formulations, such as liposomal curcumin or curcumin bound to phospholipids, to increase bioavailability. These are especially useful for those seeking maximum therapeutic effects.

Turmeric can be added to foods, teas, or taken in supplement form (curcumin extract capsules), with supplements generally providing the highest concentration of curcumin.

Dosage Guidelines and Potential Side Effects

- **Dosage**: For general cognitive support and anti-inflammatory benefits, doses typically range from 500 mg to 2,000 mg of curcumin per day, often divided into two doses. Many studies use doses of around 1,000 mg per day for cognitive effects. Always follow specific product guidelines.

- **Potential Side Effects**: Curcumin is generally well tolerated, but high doses may cause digestive issues such as nausea, diarrhea, or stomach cramps in some people. Taking it with food can help minimize these effects. Additionally, because curcumin has mild blood-thinning effects, people on anticoagulant medications should consult a healthcare provider before starting curcumin supplements.

In summary, curcumin is a powerful natural compound with significant benefits for brain health, focus, and mental clarity, particularly when taken with black pepper or fats for optimal absorption. As an anti-inflammatory and antioxidant, curcumin can support cognitive function over time, making it a valuable supplement for those looking to enhance focus and protect against cognitive decline.

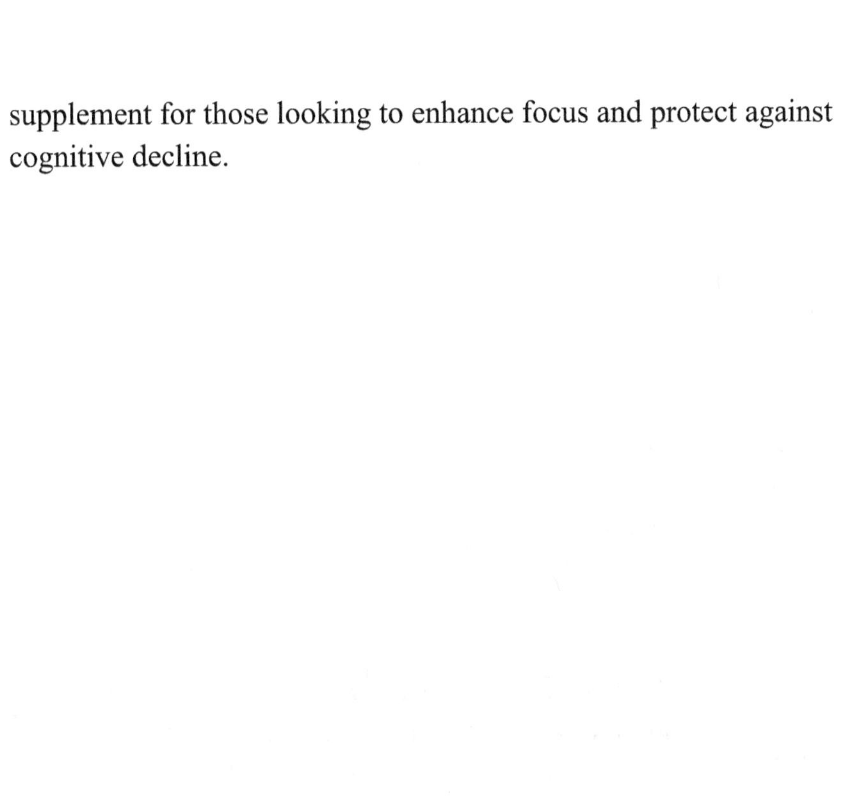

7. Magnesium: The Essential Mineral for Neurological Health

Magnesium is a true powerhouse when it comes to supporting overall health, and its role in neurological function is particularly noteworthy. Let's uncover the various forms of magnesium, their specific benefits, and how they contribute to a healthy mind.

Exploring the Diverse Forms of Magnesium:

Magnesium L-Threonate: This form of magnesium is a true champion for brain health. Its unique ability to cross the blood-brain barrier makes it highly effective in supporting cognitive function. Studies suggest that magnesium L-threonate may enhance memory, learning, and overall brain performance.

Magnesium Citrate: Known for its excellent bioavailability, magnesium citrate is a popular choice for those seeking to optimize their magnesium intake. It's particularly beneficial for supporting digestive health and promoting regular bowel movements.

Magnesium Glycinate: Magnesium glycinate is a highly absorbable form of magnesium that is gentle on the stomach. It's often recommended for individuals with sensitive digestive systems and is known to support muscle and nerve function.

Magnesium Malate: This form of magnesium combines the benefits of magnesium with the organic compound malic acid. It's believed to support energy production and is often used by individuals with chronic fatigue syndrome or fibromyalgia.

Magnesium Taurate: A combination of magnesium and the amino acid taurine, this form of magnesium is known for its calming effects on the nervous system. It may help reduce anxiety and promote a sense of relaxation, making it a popular choice for stress management.

Magnesium Chloride: Derived from ancient seabeds, magnesium chloride is a highly absorbable form of magnesium. It's often used topically in the form of magnesium oil or applied transdermally for quick absorption.

The Neurological Benefits of Magnesium:

Magnesium plays a crucial role in supporting neurological health in several ways:

Neurotransmitter Regulation: Magnesium helps regulate the release and uptake of neurotransmitters, ensuring proper communication between nerve cells. This is vital for maintaining a healthy nervous system and optimal cognitive function.

Anxiety and Stress Management: Magnesium's calming effects on the nervous system make it an excellent natural remedy for reducing anxiety and promoting relaxation. It helps regulate stress hormones like cortisol, contributing to a sense of calm and well-being.

Cognitive Function: Various forms of magnesium, particularly magnesium L-threonate, have been shown to enhance cognitive function, improve memory, and support overall brain health.

Recommended Intake and Precautions:

The recommended daily intake of magnesium varies based on age, gender, and individual health needs. It's always best to consult with a healthcare professional to determine the appropriate dosage for your specific requirements. Now Brand Capsules provide 400mg per serving of a blend of Magnesium Oxide, Citrate, and Aspertate where it is suggested to take 1 capsule daily.

While magnesium is generally well-tolerated, excessive intake can lead to side effects such as diarrhea, nausea, and abdominal discomfort. Individuals with kidney problems should exercise caution and seek professional advice before supplementing with magnesium.

In conclusion, magnesium is an essential mineral with a diverse range of forms, each offering unique benefits for neurological health. Whether you're seeking to support cognitive function, manage anxiety, or promote overall brain health, there's a form of magnesium that can help you achieve your wellness goals. As always, it's best to consult with a healthcare professional to ensure you're taking the right form and dosage for your individual needs.

8. Vitamin D: The Sunshine Vitamin

Vitamin D, often referred to as the "sunshine vitamin," plays a crucial role in maintaining overall health and well-being. Its impact extends beyond bone health, as it also influences cognitive function, mood regulation, and energy levels. Here's a comprehensive look at the role of Vitamin D in cognitive health:

Vitamin D's Role in Cognitive Function and Mood Regulation:

Vitamin D receptors are present in various areas of the brain, including those involved in cognitive function and mood regulation. Adequate Vitamin D levels are essential for optimal brain health and have been linked to improved cognitive performance, enhanced focus, and a reduced risk of cognitive decline.

Additionally, Vitamin D plays a crucial role in the production and regulation of neurotransmitters like serotonin and dopamine, which are key players in mood regulation. Low Vitamin D levels have been associated with an increased risk of depression, anxiety, and other mood disorders.

Deficiency and Its Impact on Focus and Energy Levels:

Vitamin D deficiency can have a significant impact on cognitive function and energy levels. Individuals with low Vitamin D levels often report difficulties with focus, concentration, and mental clarity. This deficiency can also lead to fatigue, low energy levels, and an overall sense of lethargy.

Research on Vitamin D's Impact on Cognitive Performance:

Numerous studies have explored the relationship between Vitamin D and cognitive function. For instance, a study published in the Journal of Alzheimer's Disease found that Vitamin D supplementation improved cognitive performance in older adults with mild cognitive impairment.

Another study, published in the journal Neurology, suggested that Vitamin D deficiency may be a risk factor for cognitive decline and dementia. The researchers found that individuals with low Vitamin D levels had a higher risk of developing cognitive impairment over time.

Optimal Levels, Recommended Dosages, and Supplementation:

The optimal Vitamin D level for cognitive health is generally considered to be between 30 ng/mL and 100 ng/mL. However, the recommended dosage for supplementation can vary based on age, health status, and individual needs.

The most natural way to obtain Vitamin D is through sunlight exposure, as the skin can synthesize Vitamin D when exposed to UVB rays. However, factors like geographical location, season, time of day, and skin pigmentation can affect Vitamin D production.

For those who have difficulty obtaining sufficient Vitamin D from sunlight, supplements are a viable option. Vitamin D supplements are available in two forms: Vitamin D2 (ergocalciferol) and Vitamin D3 (cholecalciferol). Vitamin D3 is generally considered more effective at raising and maintaining Vitamin D levels in the body.

Safety, Toxicity Risks, and Monitoring Levels:

Vitamin D is generally safe when taken at recommended dosages. However, excessive intake can lead to Vitamin D toxicity, which can cause a range of symptoms, including nausea, vomiting, poor appetite, constipation, weakness, and weight loss. In severe cases, it can lead to kidney damage and abnormal heart rhythms.

It's important to have your Vitamin D levels monitored regularly, especially if you're taking supplements. This can help ensure that you maintain optimal levels and avoid the risks associated with both deficiency and excess.

In conclusion, Vitamin D plays a vital role in cognitive function, mood regulation, and overall brain health. Maintaining adequate Vitamin D levels through sunlight exposure or supplementation can help support cognitive performance, focus, and energy levels. As with any supplement, it's essential to consult a healthcare professional to determine the appropriate dosage and monitor Vitamin D levels to ensure optimal health.

9. B-Complex Vitamins Improve Focus and Mental Clarity

The B-complex vitamins are a group of essential nutrients that play a crucial role in maintaining overall health, with a particular focus on brain function and cognitive well-being. Let's delve into the world of B vitamins, exploring their unique benefits, synergy, and impact on mental clarity and focus.

Overview of B Vitamins and Their Synergy:

The B-complex vitamins consist of eight water-soluble vitamins: thiamin (B1), riboflavin (B2), niacin (B3), pantothenic acid (B5), pyridoxine (B6), biotin (B7), folate (B9), and cobalamin (B12). These vitamins often work synergistically, meaning they enhance each other's functions and are more effective when taken together.

How Each B Vitamin Supports Brain Function:

Thiamin (B1): Thiamin is essential for the proper functioning of the nervous system. It plays a crucial role in the production of acetylcholine, a neurotransmitter involved in memory and learning.

Riboflavin (B2): Riboflavin is involved in energy production within the brain cells. It helps convert food into energy, which is vital for optimal brain function.

Niacin (B3): Niacin supports brain health by maintaining the myelin sheath, a protective covering around nerve fibers. This ensures efficient nerve impulse transmission.

Pantothenic Acid (B5): B5 is involved in the production of neurotransmitters and is essential for proper nerve function.

Pyridoxine (B6): B6 is crucial for the synthesis of several neurotransmitters, including serotonin, norepinephrine, and GABA. These neurotransmitters play a key role in mood regulation, cognitive function, and sleep.

Biotin (B7): While biotin's role in brain health is less understood, it is essential for energy production and the metabolism of fatty acids, which are crucial for brain function.

Folate (B9): Folate is involved in the synthesis of DNA and RNA, making it essential for proper brain development and function. It also plays a role in the production of neurotransmitters.

Cobalamin (B12): B12 is vital for the maintenance of nerve cells and the production of myelin. It also helps regulate mood and cognitive function by supporting the synthesis of neurotransmitters.

Benefits for Energy Production, Focus, and Mental Clarity:

The B-complex vitamins are often referred to as the "energy vitamins" due to their crucial role in energy production. They help convert food into energy, ensuring the brain and body have the fuel they need for optimal performance.

Additionally, B vitamins support focus and mental clarity by maintaining healthy nerve function, regulating neurotransmitter production, and promoting efficient brain metabolism.

Research on B Complex and Cognitive Health:

Numerous studies have highlighted the positive impact of B vitamins on cognitive health. For instance, a study published in the journal Neurology found that higher intakes of B vitamins, particularly B6, B12, and folate, were associated with a reduced risk of cognitive decline and dementia.

Another study, published in the journal Nutritional Neuroscience, suggested that B-vitamin supplementation may improve cognitive performance in older adults, particularly in areas of memory and executive function.

Dosage Recommendations and Ideal Forms:

The recommended daily intake of B vitamins can vary based on age, gender, and individual health needs. It's generally recommended to obtain B vitamins from a balanced diet that includes a variety of whole foods, such as meat, fish, eggs, dairy, legumes, and leafy green vegetables.

For those who require supplementation, methylated forms of B vitamins, such as methylcobalamin (B12) and methylfolate (B9), are often recommended. These forms are more easily absorbed and utilized by the body, especially in individuals with certain genetic variations that affect their ability to convert traditional forms of B vitamins.

Precautions and Possible Side Effects:

B vitamins are generally considered safe when taken at recommended dosages. However, excessive intake of certain B vitamins, particularly niacin (B3), can lead to flushing, itching, and gastrointestinal upset.

It's important to note that some B vitamins, such as B6 and B12, can interact with certain medications. Always consult with a healthcare professional before starting any new supplement regimen, especially if you have underlying health conditions or are taking medications.

In conclusion, the B-complex vitamins are a powerful group of nutrients that work together to support brain function, energy production, and mental clarity. Maintaining adequate levels of B vitamins through a balanced diet and, if necessary, targeted supplementation, can contribute to optimal cognitive health and well-being. As always, it's best to consult with a healthcare professional to determine the most appropriate dosage and form of B vitamins for your individual needs.

10. Saffron: A Spice for Cognitive Enhancement

Saffron, derived from the flower of the Crocus sativus plant, is a precious spice known for its vibrant color, distinct flavor, and numerous health benefits. It has been used for centuries in traditional medicine and culinary practices, particularly in the Middle East, India, and Europe. Saffron's unique properties and potential cognitive benefits have made it a subject of interest in modern scientific research.

Neuroprotective and Cognitive-Enhancing Properties:

Saffron contains a variety of bioactive compounds, including crocin, crocetin, and safranal, which are responsible for its unique properties. These compounds have been studied for their potential neuroprotective effects and their ability to enhance cognitive function.

Neuroprotection: Saffron's active components have shown promising results in protecting brain cells from damage caused by oxidative stress and inflammation. This neuroprotective effect may contribute to the prevention of cognitive decline and neurodegenerative diseases.

Cognitive Enhancement: Research suggests that saffron can improve various aspects of cognitive function, including memory, attention, and focus. It may enhance learning abilities, information processing, and overall mental performance.

Research on Saffron's Impact:

Numerous studies have explored the impact of saffron on cognitive health and mood. Here are some key findings:

Mood Enhancement: Saffron has been found to have antidepressant-like effects. A study published in the Journal of Affective Disorders showed that saffron supplementation improved symptoms of depression in adults. It is believed that saffron's active compounds modulate neurotransmitter systems, leading to improved mood and reduced anxiety.

Focus and Attention: Research indicates that saffron can enhance focus and attention. A randomized controlled trial published in the Journal of Clinical Pharmacy and Therapeutics found that saffron supplementation improved attention and cognitive performance in healthy adults.

Memory Improvement: Saffron's potential to enhance memory has been a subject of interest. A study in the Journal of Clinical Psychopharmacology reported that saffron extract improved verbal and visual memory in older adults. This suggests that saffron may have a positive impact on age-related cognitive decline.

Suggested Dosages and Considerations:

When using saffron as a supplement, it is important to consider the following:

Dosage: The recommended dosage of saffron can vary depending on the form and purpose of use. For cognitive enhancement, a typical dosage ranges from 30-100 mg per day.

However, it is best to consult a healthcare professional for personalized advice.

Form: Saffron is available in various forms, including capsules, extracts, and threads. The form chosen may depend on individual preferences and the intended use.

Quality: Opt for high-quality saffron from reputable sources to ensure purity and potency.

Duration: Saffron supplements are generally safe for short-term use. However, long-term use should be discussed with a healthcare provider to ensure optimal benefits and avoid potential side effects.

Potential Side Effects and Interactions:

Saffron is generally considered safe when used appropriately. However, some individuals may experience mild side effects, such as headaches, dizziness, or allergic reactions. It is important to be aware of the following:

Allergic Reactions: Some people may be allergic to saffron. If any signs of an allergic reaction occur, such as skin rash, itching, or difficulty breathing, discontinue use and seek medical advice.

Drug Interactions: Saffron may interact with certain medications, especially those affecting the central nervous system. It is crucial to inform your healthcare provider about any medications you are taking before starting saffron supplementation.

Pregnancy and Breastfeeding: Pregnant and breastfeeding women should consult their healthcare providers before using saffron supplements, as there is limited research on its safety during these periods.

In conclusion, saffron offers a natural approach to enhancing cognitive function, mood, and focus. Its neuroprotective properties and potential to improve memory and attention make it an intriguing supplement for those seeking to optimize their brain health. As with any supplement, it is essential to use saffron responsibly and consult healthcare professionals for personalized guidance.

11. Panax Ginseng: An Adaptogenic Herb for Cognitive Enhancement

Panax Ginseng, often referred to as Korean Ginseng, is a renowned herb with a long history of traditional use, particularly in East Asian cultures. It belongs to the genus Panax, known for its adaptogenic properties, which enable the body to adapt and respond to stress more effectively. The root of Panax Ginseng has been utilized for centuries to promote overall well-being and enhance various physiological functions.

Enhancing Focus and Energy

One of the key benefits associated with Panax Ginseng is its ability to support focus, energy levels, and cognitive function. This adaptogenic herb contains active compounds, including ginsenosides, which are believed to be responsible for its cognitive-enhancing effects. Ginsenosides have been studied for their potential to improve mental performance, especially in tasks requiring sustained attention and concentration.

Cognitive Function and Brain Health

Panax Ginseng's impact on cognitive function extends beyond enhanced focus. Research suggests that this herb may contribute to improved memory, learning abilities, and overall brain health. Its adaptogenic properties help modulate the body's response to stress, which is crucial for maintaining optimal cognitive function. Additionally, Panax Ginseng has been found to possess antioxidant effects, which can protect brain cells from oxidative damage, a key factor in cognitive decline.

Evidence on Cognitive Performance

Numerous studies have investigated the effects of Panax Ginseng on cognitive performance, with promising results. A systematic review and meta-analysis published in the Journal of Ethnopharmacology concluded that Panax Ginseng supplementation led to significant improvements in cognitive function, particularly in areas of attention, processing speed, and working memory. Another study, published in the Journal of Psychopharmacology, found that Panax Ginseng extract improved cognitive performance and reduced mental fatigue in healthy young adults.

Recommended Dosages and Considerations

The recommended dosage of Panax Ginseng can vary depending on the form and concentration of the supplement. Generally, it is advised to start with lower doses and gradually increase as needed. For standardized Panax Ginseng extracts, a common dosage range is 200-400 mg per day, taken in divided doses. It is essential to consult with a healthcare professional, especially if you have any underlying health conditions or are taking medications, as Panax Ginseng may interact with certain drugs.

Precautions and Side Effects

While Panax Ginseng is generally considered safe for most individuals, it is important to be aware of potential side effects and precautions. Some people may experience mild gastrointestinal symptoms, such as upset stomach or diarrhea, when taking Panax Ginseng. It is also not recommended for individuals with certain medical conditions, such as autoimmune disorders or bleeding disorders, without medical supervision. Additionally, Panax Ginseng may interact with blood-thinning medications, so caution is advised. As with any supplement, it is best to consult a healthcare provider before starting Panax Ginseng supplementation.

12. Chia Seeds: A Nutritious Source of Omega-3s for Brain Health

Omega-3 Fatty Acids and Brain Health

Chia seeds are an excellent natural source of Omega-3 fatty acids, which are essential for maintaining optimal brain health and cognitive function. Omega-3s, particularly docosahexaenoic acid (DHA) and eicosapentaenoic acid (EPA), play a crucial role in supporting the structure and function of the brain. These fatty acids are integral components of brain cell membranes and are involved in various neurological processes.

Cognitive Function and Focus

The Omega-3 fatty acids found in chia seeds have been extensively studied for their positive impact on cognitive function. Research suggests that adequate intake of Omega-3s is associated with improved memory, learning abilities, and overall cognitive performance. These fatty acids help maintain the fluidity of cell membranes, facilitating efficient communication between brain cells and enhancing cognitive processes.

Research on Omega-3s and Brain Health

Numerous scientific studies have investigated the relationship between Omega-3 fatty acid intake and brain health. A systematic review and meta-analysis published in the Journal of the American Medical Association found that higher intakes of Omega-3s, particularly DHA, were associated with a reduced risk of cognitive decline and improved cognitive performance in older adults. Another study, published in the American Journal of Clinical Nutrition, reported that Omega-3 supplementation led to significant improvements in cognitive function and reduced cognitive decline in individuals with mild cognitive impairment.

Incorporating Chia Seeds for Brain Support

Chia seeds are a convenient and versatile way to incorporate Omega-3 fatty acids into your diet. They can be easily added to a variety of dishes, such as smoothies, oatmeal, yogurt, or baked goods. To ensure optimal brain support, aim for a daily intake of at least 2-3 tablespoons of chia seeds. Chia seeds can also be soaked in water or milk to create a gel-like substance, which can be used as a healthy alternative to eggs in baking or as a thickener in sauces and dressings.

Potential Side Effects and Considerations

Chia seeds are generally well-tolerated and considered safe for most individuals. However, as with any food, some people may experience mild gastrointestinal symptoms, such as bloating or gas, when consuming chia seeds in large amounts. It is important to start with smaller portions and gradually increase intake to assess individual tolerance. Additionally, individuals with a history of swallowing difficulties or those taking certain medications should consult with a healthcare professional before significantly increasing their chia seed intake.

In conclusion, chia seeds are a nutritious and convenient source of Omega-3 fatty acids, which are essential for brain health and cognitive function. Incorporating chia seeds into your diet can be a simple and effective way to support optimal brain function and overall well-being.

13. Cat's Claw: A Traditional Herb with Potential Cognitive Benefits

Traditional Use and Introduction

Cat's Claw, scientifically known as Uncaria tomentosa, is a tropical vine native to the Amazon rainforest. It has a long history of traditional use by indigenous communities in South America, particularly for its potential medicinal properties. The inner bark and root of Cat's Claw have been utilized for centuries to support overall health and well-being. Its name derives from the small, curved thorns resembling a cat's claw, which are a distinctive feature of the plant.

Cognitive Benefits and Neuroprotection

Cat's Claw has gained attention for its potential cognitive benefits and neuroprotective properties. Research suggests that this herb may help support focus, memory, and overall cognitive function. It contains a variety of bioactive compounds, including alkaloids and antioxidants, which are believed to contribute to its cognitive-enhancing effects.

The neuroprotective properties of Cat's Claw are particularly intriguing. Studies have indicated that certain compounds in Cat's Claw may help protect brain cells from damage caused by oxidative stress and inflammation. This neuroprotective action could potentially slow down cognitive decline and support brain health as we age.

Research on Focus and Cognitive Function

Several studies have explored the impact of Cat's Claw on cognitive performance. A randomized, double-blind, placebo-controlled trial published in the Journal of Alternative and Complementary Medicine found that Cat's Claw supplementation led to significant improvements in attention and cognitive processing speed. Another study, published in the Journal of Ethnopharmacology, reported that Cat's Claw extract improved memory and learning abilities in animal models.

Suggested Dosages and Considerations

The recommended dosage of Cat's Claw can vary depending on the form and concentration of the supplement. For standardized Cat's Claw extracts, a common dosage range is 250-500 mg per day, taken in divided doses. It is advisable to start with a lower dose and gradually increase as needed. Cat's Claw is available in various forms, including capsules, tablets, and tinctures.

It is important to note that Cat's Claw may interact with certain medications, particularly those that affect the immune system. Individuals with autoimmune disorders or those taking immunosuppressive drugs should exercise caution and consult with a healthcare professional before using Cat's Claw. Cat's Claw is also used for Lyme Disease, dosages and preparations may be found on Dr. Rawls website and in his books, based on herbalist Stephen Buhner's Research.

Potential Side Effects and Interactions

Cat's Claw is generally considered safe for most individuals when used appropriately. However, as with any herbal supplement, some people may experience mild side effects, such as gastrointestinal discomfort or allergic reactions. It is recommended to start with a low dose and monitor for any adverse reactions.

Additionally, Cat's Claw may interact with certain medications, including blood thinners and immunosuppressants. It is crucial to consult with a healthcare provider, especially if you have any underlying health conditions or are taking medications, to ensure safe and effective use of Cat's Claw.

In conclusion, Cat's Claw is a traditional herb with potential cognitive benefits and neuroprotective properties. While more research is needed to fully understand its mechanisms of action, the existing evidence suggests that Cat's Claw may be a valuable addition to a brain-supportive regimen. As with any herbal supplement, it is essential to use Cat's Claw under the guidance of a healthcare professional to ensure safety and effectiveness.

14. Shilajit: An Ancient Adaptogen for Cognitive Enhancement

Shilajit is a natural substance with a long history of use in traditional Ayurvedic medicine. It is a dark, sticky resin found in the rocks of the Himalayas and other mountainous regions. In Ayurveda, Shilajit is considered a powerful rejuvenating and adaptogenic substance, often referred to as "conqueror of mountains and destroyer of weakness." It has been utilized for centuries to promote overall health, vitality, and cognitive function.

Adaptogenic and Cognitive-Enhancing Properties

Shilajit is renowned for its adaptogenic properties, which enable the body to adapt and respond to stress more effectively. It contains a unique combination of fulvic acid, humic acid, and various minerals, including iron and trace elements. These components are believed to contribute to its cognitive-enhancing effects. Shilajit has been studied for its potential to improve focus, memory, and overall cognitive performance.

Antioxidant Effects and Brain Health

One of the key benefits of Shilajit is its potent antioxidant activity. It contains a high concentration of antioxidants, which can help protect brain cells from oxidative damage. Oxidative stress is a major contributor to cognitive decline and various neurological disorders. By neutralizing free radicals, Shilajit's antioxidants may support brain health and promote optimal cognitive function.

Evidence on Cognitive Performance

Several studies have investigated the impact of Shilajit on cognitive performance, with promising results. A randomized, double-blind, placebo-controlled trial published in the Journal of Dietary Supplements found that Shilajit supplementation led to significant improvements in memory and cognitive function in healthy adults. Another study, published in the Journal of Ethnopharmacology, reported that Shilajit extract improved cognitive performance and reduced mental fatigue in individuals with mild cognitive impairment.

Recommended Dosages and Considerations

The recommended dosage of Shilajit can vary depending on the form and concentration of the supplement. For standardized Shilajit extracts, a common dosage range is 200-400 mg per day, taken in divided doses. It is advisable to start with a lower dose and gradually increase as needed. Shilajit is available in various forms, including capsules, tablets, and powders.

It is important to note that Shilajit may contain small amounts of heavy metals, such as lead and mercury, due to its natural source. Reputable manufacturers ensure that their Shilajit products are tested and meet safety standards. It is recommended to choose high-quality, purified Shilajit supplements to minimize the risk of heavy metal exposure.

Precautions and Potential Side Effects

Shilajit is generally considered safe for most individuals when used appropriately. However, as with any supplement, some people may experience mild side effects, such as gastrointestinal discomfort or allergic reactions. It is advisable to start with a low dose and monitor for any adverse reactions.

Individuals with certain medical conditions, such as kidney or liver disease, should exercise caution and consult with a healthcare professional before using Shilajit. Additionally, pregnant and breastfeeding women are advised to avoid Shilajit due to a lack of sufficient safety data.

In conclusion, Shilajit is an ancient adaptogen with potential cognitive-enhancing and brain-supportive properties. Its adaptogenic nature, antioxidant effects, and traditional use in Ayurveda make it an intriguing natural substance for promoting cognitive health. As with any supplement, it is essential to use Shilajit under the guidance of a healthcare professional to ensure safety and effectiveness.

15. N-Acetyl Cysteine (NAC): A Versatile Supplement for Weight Loss and Cognitive Support

N-Acetyl Cysteine (NAC) is a derivative of the amino acid cysteine and is a popular dietary supplement known for its diverse health benefits. It has gained attention for its potential to support weight loss and enhance cognitive function, making it a versatile supplement for overall well-being.

Weight Loss Support

NAC has shown promise in aiding weight loss efforts. One of its key mechanisms of action is its ability to support the body's natural detoxification processes. NAC helps increase glutathione levels, a powerful antioxidant that plays a crucial role in detoxifying the body and promoting overall health. By supporting detoxification, NAC may contribute to weight loss by reducing inflammation and improving metabolic function.

Additionally, NAC has been studied for its potential to reduce appetite and promote satiety. It may help regulate hormones involved in hunger and fullness, leading to a decreased desire for excessive food intake. This appetite-regulating effect can be beneficial for individuals aiming to manage their weight and maintain a healthy diet.

Enhancing Focus and Cognitive Function

Beyond its weight loss benefits, NAC is well-known for its positive impact on cognitive function. It is a precursor to glutathione, an essential antioxidant that protects brain cells from oxidative damage. By supporting glutathione production, NAC helps maintain optimal brain health and cognitive performance.

Research suggests that NAC may improve focus, attention, and overall cognitive function. It has been studied in individuals with cognitive impairments, such as those with mild cognitive decline or attention-deficit/hyperactivity disorder (ADHD), showing promising results in enhancing cognitive performance. NAC's ability to support brain health and cognitive function makes it a valuable supplement for individuals seeking to optimize their mental clarity and focus.

Recommended Dosages and Considerations

The recommended dosage of NAC can vary depending on the intended use and individual needs. For weight loss support, a common dosage range is 600-1200 mg per day, taken in divided doses. For cognitive enhancement, a higher dosage of 1200-2400 mg per day may be recommended. It is important to start with a lower dose and gradually increase as needed, under the guidance of a healthcare professional.

NAC is generally considered safe for most individuals when used appropriately. However, as with any supplement, it is essential to consult with a healthcare provider, especially if you have any underlying health conditions or are taking medications. NAC may interact with certain medications, so caution is advised.

Precautions and Potential Side Effects

While NAC is generally well-tolerated, some individuals may experience mild side effects, such as nausea, vomiting, or gastrointestinal discomfort. These side effects are typically dose-dependent and can be minimized by starting with lower doses and gradually increasing.

It is important to note that NAC should not be used as a sole treatment for any medical condition, including obesity or cognitive impairments. It should be used as a supportive supplement under the guidance of a healthcare professional.

In conclusion, N-Acetyl Cysteine (NAC) is a versatile supplement with potential benefits for weight loss and cognitive support. Its ability to support detoxification, regulate appetite, and enhance cognitive function makes it a valuable addition to a healthy lifestyle. As with any supplement, it is crucial to use NAC responsibly and consult with a healthcare provider for personalized advice and guidance.

16. Garlic and Chlorella: Natural Allies for Cognitive Enhancement and Detoxification

Garlic (Allium sativum) and Chlorella (Chlorella pyrenoidosa) are two natural substances that have gained attention for their potential benefits in supporting cognitive function, focus, and detoxification. These powerful allies have been studied for their individual and combined effects, offering promising results for overall health and well-being.

Cognitive Benefits and Focus

Garlic

Garlic is renowned for its cognitive-enhancing properties. It contains a variety of compounds, including allicin and S-allyl cysteine, which are believed to contribute to its positive effects on brain health. Research suggests that garlic may improve memory, learning abilities, and overall cognitive performance. Its antioxidant and anti-inflammatory properties help protect brain cells from damage and support optimal cognitive function.

Chlorella

Chlorella, a single-celled green algae, is a nutritional powerhouse packed with essential nutrients. It is rich in chlorophyll, amino acids, vitamins, and minerals, making it an excellent food for overall health. In terms of cognition, Chlorella has been studied for its potential to enhance focus and mental clarity. Its high antioxidant content helps reduce oxidative stress in the brain, which is associated with improved cognitive function.

Detoxification and Heavy Metal Elimination

Garlic

Garlic has long been recognized for its detoxifying properties. It contains sulfur-containing compounds, such as allicin, which have been shown to support the body's natural detoxification processes. Garlic helps stimulate liver function, promote the elimination of toxins, and enhance the body's ability to remove heavy metals. Its sulfur compounds also play a role in supporting the body's natural defense mechanisms against environmental toxins.

Chlorella

Chlorella is a potent detoxifier, particularly effective in eliminating heavy metals from the body. It has a unique cell wall structure that binds to heavy metals, such as lead, mercury, and cadmium, facilitating their removal from the body. Chlorella's ability to chelate heavy metals makes it a valuable tool for detoxification and supporting overall health.

Research Insights from Dr. Dietrich Klinghardt

Dr. Dietrich Klinghardt, a renowned physician and expert in integrative medicine, has conducted extensive research on the benefits of garlic and chlorella. He has highlighted their potential in supporting cognitive function and detoxification:

"Garlic and Chlorella are two of the most powerful natural substances for supporting brain health and detoxification. Garlic's sulfur compounds and Chlorella's unique cell structure make them excellent allies in the fight against cognitive decline and environmental toxins. When used together, they offer a synergistic effect, enhancing their individual benefits."

Dr. Klinghardt has also emphasized the importance of proper preparation and sourcing of garlic and chlorella to maximize their therapeutic effects. He recommends using high-quality, organic, and properly processed forms of these natural substances to ensure optimal results.

Recommended Usage and Considerations

To experience the cognitive and detoxification benefits of garlic and chlorella, it is recommended to incorporate them into your diet or consider supplement forms. Garlic can be consumed raw, cooked, or in supplement form, while Chlorella is typically available as a supplement in tablet or powder form.

It is important to start with moderate doses and gradually increase as tolerated. Garlic and Chlorella may have mild side effects, such as gastrointestinal discomfort, especially when consumed in large amounts. It is advisable to consult with a healthcare professional, especially if you have any underlying health conditions or are taking medications.

In conclusion, Garlic and Chlorella offer a natural and effective approach to supporting cognitive function, focus, and detoxification. Their individual and combined benefits, supported by research and insights from experts like Dr. Dietrich Klinghardt, make them valuable additions to a holistic health regimen. As with any supplement, it is essential to use them responsibly and seek professional guidance for personalized recommendations.

17. Gotu Kola: An Ancient Herb for Energy and Focus

Gotu Kola, scientifically known as Centella Asiatica, is an ancient herb that has been used for centuries in traditional medicine systems, particularly in Ayurveda and traditional Chinese medicine. It is native to Southeast Asia and has gained recognition for its potential benefits in enhancing energy levels and cognitive function.

Energy Boosting Properties

Gotu Kola is renowned for its energizing effects on the body and mind. It contains active compounds called triterpenoid saponins, which are believed to be responsible for its energizing properties. These saponins have been studied for their ability to improve blood circulation, enhance oxygen delivery to cells, and support overall energy production.

By promoting better blood flow, Gotu Kola can help increase oxygen and nutrient delivery to the brain and other organs, leading to improved energy levels and mental clarity. Its energizing effects can be particularly beneficial for individuals experiencing fatigue, mental exhaustion, or low energy levels.

Focus and Cognitive Enhancement

In addition to its energizing properties, Gotu Kola is known for its positive impact on cognitive function and focus. It has been traditionally used to enhance memory, concentration, and overall mental performance.

Research suggests that Gotu Kola may improve brain health by promoting the growth and repair of neurons. It contains compounds that have neuroprotective properties, helping to protect brain cells from damage and supporting their optimal functioning. This can lead to improved focus, enhanced learning abilities, and better cognitive performance.

Potential Benefits for Brain Health

Gotu Kola's benefits extend beyond energy and focus. It has been studied for its potential role in supporting brain health and reducing the risk of cognitive decline. Some studies suggest that Gotu Kola may have anti-inflammatory and antioxidant effects, which can help protect the brain from oxidative stress and inflammation, both of which are associated with cognitive impairment.

Furthermore, Gotu Kola has been found to modulate neurotransmitter levels, particularly acetylcholine, which plays a crucial role in memory and cognitive processes. By regulating neurotransmitter balance, Gotu Kola may contribute to improved cognitive function and overall brain health.

Weight Loss

While Gotu Kola is primarily associated with cognitive benefits, it may also have a positive impact on weight loss. Some studies indicate that Gotu Kola can help reduce inflammation, which is often linked to obesity and metabolic disorders. Its potential to improve blood circulation and support healthy digestion may contribute to a holistic approach to weight management.

How to Incorporate Gotu Kola

Gotu Kola can be consumed in various forms to reap its energizing and cognitive-enhancing benefits:

Tea: Brew Gotu Kola leaves or use pre-made Gotu Kola tea bags. Enjoy a cup of warm tea to relax and energize.

Capsules or Tablets: Gotu Kola supplements are widely available in capsule or tablet form. Follow the recommended dosage instructions on the product label.

Tinctures: Gotu Kola tinctures can be added to water or juice for a convenient way to consume the herb.

Fresh or Dried Leaves: If you have access to fresh Gotu Kola leaves, you can add them to salads, smoothies, or soups. Dried leaves can also be used in cooking or brewing tea.

It's important to note that while Gotu Kola is generally considered safe, it may interact with certain medications or have potential side effects in high doses. It is always advisable to consult with a healthcare professional before incorporating Gotu Kola or any herbal supplement into your routine, especially if you have any underlying health conditions.

In conclusion, Gotu Kola is an ancient herb with potential benefits for energy, focus, and brain health. Its energizing properties, cognitive-enhancing effects, and potential role in supporting brain health make it a valuable addition to a holistic approach to well-being. As with any herbal remedy, moderation and consultation with a healthcare professional are key to ensuring safe and effective use.

18. Rhodiola Rosea: An Adaptogenic Herb for Energy and Focus

Rhodiola Rosea, also known as Arctic Root or Golden Root, is a powerful adaptogenic herb that has been used for centuries in traditional medicine systems, particularly in Scandinavia and Siberia. It has gained recognition for its ability to enhance energy levels, improve mental performance, and promote overall well-being.

Energy Boosting Properties

Rhodiola Rosea is renowned for its energizing effects, making it a popular choice for individuals seeking a natural boost in energy and stamina. It contains active compounds called rosavins and salidrosides, which are believed to be responsible for its energizing properties.

These compounds work synergistically to enhance energy production in the body by improving mitochondrial function and increasing the efficiency of cellular energy metabolism. Rhodiola Rosea can help combat fatigue, increase physical endurance, and promote a sense of vitality and vigor.

Focus and Cognitive Enhancement

In addition to its energizing effects, Rhodiola Rosea is known for its positive impact on cognitive function and focus. It has been studied for its ability to enhance mental performance, improve concentration, and reduce mental fatigue.

Research suggests that Rhodiola Rosea may improve cognitive function by increasing the availability of neurotransmitters, such as serotonin and dopamine, in the brain. It also has neuroprotective properties, helping to protect brain cells from damage and supporting their optimal functioning.

Rhodiola Rosea has been found to enhance memory, attention span, and overall mental clarity. Its adaptogenic properties help the body adapt to stress, improving resilience and cognitive performance under challenging conditions.

Stress Relief and Mood Enhancement

Rhodiola Rosea is not only beneficial for energy and focus but also for stress relief and mood enhancement. It has been traditionally used to promote emotional well-being and reduce symptoms of anxiety and depression.

The adaptogenic properties of Rhodiola Rosea help modulate the body's stress response, reducing the negative impact of stress on both physical and mental health. It can help individuals cope with stress more effectively, improve mood, and promote a sense of calm and balance.

How to Incorporate Rhodiola Rosea

Rhodiola Rosea can be consumed in various forms to harness its energizing and cognitive-enhancing benefits:

Supplements: Rhodiola Rosea supplements are widely available in capsule or tablet form. Follow the recommended dosage instructions on the product label.

Tea: Brew Rhodiola Rosea tea using the dried root or pre-made tea bags. Enjoy a cup of warm tea to relax and energize.

Tinctures: Rhodiola Rosea tinctures can be added to water or juice for a convenient way to consume the herb.

Fresh or Dried Root: If you have access to fresh or dried Rhodiola Rosea root, you can add it to smoothies, soups, or stews.

It's important to note that while Rhodiola Rosea is generally considered safe, it may interact with certain medications or have potential side effects in high doses. It is always advisable to consult with a healthcare professional before incorporating Rhodiola Rosea or any herbal supplement into your routine, especially if you have any underlying health conditions.

In conclusion, Rhodiola Rosea is a powerful adaptogenic herb that offers a natural solution for enhancing energy levels, improving cognitive function, and promoting overall well-being. Its energizing, cognitive-enhancing, and stress-relieving properties make it a valuable addition to a holistic approach to health and vitality. As with any herbal remedy, moderation and consultation with a healthcare professional are essential for safe and effective use.

19. Ashwagandha: An Ancient Herb for Energy, Focus, and Stress Relief

Ashwagandha, scientifically known as Withania somnifera, is an ancient herb that has been used for thousands of years in traditional Ayurvedic medicine. It is native to India and has gained recognition for its numerous health benefits, particularly in enhancing energy levels, improving focus, and promoting stress relief.

Energy Boosting Properties

Ashwagandha is renowned for its ability to boost energy and combat fatigue. It contains active compounds called withanolides, which are believed to be responsible for its energizing effects. These compounds work by supporting the body's natural energy production processes and enhancing overall vitality.

By reducing oxidative stress and supporting mitochondrial function, Ashwagandha helps optimize energy metabolism. It can increase stamina, improve physical performance, and provide a natural boost in energy levels, making it an excellent choice for individuals seeking a sustainable source of energy.

Focus and Cognitive Enhancement

In addition to its energizing properties, Ashwagandha is known for its positive impact on cognitive function and focus. It has been traditionally used to enhance memory, concentration, and overall mental performance.

Research suggests that Ashwagandha may improve cognitive function by reducing stress-induced cognitive impairment. It helps modulate neurotransmitter levels, particularly acetylcholine, which plays a crucial role in memory and learning. Ashwagandha's adaptogenic properties also contribute to improved focus and mental clarity.

Stress Relief and Anxiety Reduction

One of the most well-known benefits of Ashwagandha is its ability to promote stress relief and reduce anxiety. It has been extensively studied for its anxiolytic and adaptogenic properties.

Ashwagandha helps regulate the body's stress response by modulating the hypothalamic-pituitary-adrenal (HPA) axis, a key component of the stress response system. It can lower cortisol levels, a hormone associated with stress, and promote a sense of calm and relaxation. Ashwagandha's anxiolytic effects can help individuals manage stress, improve mood, and enhance overall well-being.

How to Incorporate Ashwagandha

Ashwagandha can be consumed in various forms to harness its energizing, cognitive-enhancing, and stress-relieving benefits:

Supplements: Ashwagandha supplements are widely available in capsule or tablet form. Follow the recommended dosage instructions on the product label.

Tea: Brew Ashwagandha tea using the dried root or pre-made tea bags. Enjoy a cup of warm tea to relax and energize.

Tinctures: Ashwagandha tinctures can be added to water or juice for a convenient way to consume the herb.

Powder: Ashwagandha powder can be mixed into smoothies, yogurt, or oatmeal for a nutritional boost.

It's important to note that while Ashwagandha is generally considered safe, it may interact with certain medications or have potential side effects in high doses. It is always advisable to consult with a healthcare professional before incorporating Ashwagandha or any herbal supplement into your routine, especially if you have any underlying health conditions.

In conclusion, Ashwagandha is a powerful ancient herb that offers a holistic approach to enhancing energy levels, improving cognitive function, and promoting stress relief. Its energizing, cognitive-enhancing, and anxiolytic properties make it a valuable addition to a natural and balanced lifestyle. As with any herbal remedy, moderation and consultation with a healthcare professional are key to ensuring safe and effective use.

20. Ginkgo Biloba: An Ancient Herb for Cognitive Enhancement and Energy

Ginkgo Biloba is an ancient herb that has been used for centuries in traditional Chinese medicine and is one of the oldest living tree species. It is renowned for its potential to enhance cognitive function, improve energy levels, and promote overall brain health.

Cognitive Enhancement

Ginkgo Biloba is widely recognized for its positive impact on cognitive performance. It contains unique compounds called ginkgo flavone glycosides and terpene lactones, which are believed to be responsible for its cognitive-enhancing effects.

These compounds work by improving blood flow to the brain, enhancing oxygen and nutrient delivery to brain cells. Ginkgo Biloba has been shown to increase mental alertness, improve memory, and enhance overall cognitive function. It may also help protect brain cells from damage caused by free radicals, reducing the risk of cognitive decline.

Energy Boost and Mental Fatigue Reduction

In addition to its cognitive benefits, Ginkgo Biloba is known for its ability to boost energy levels and reduce mental fatigue. It can help improve focus and concentration, making it beneficial for individuals who experience mental exhaustion or have demanding cognitive tasks.

By enhancing blood circulation and oxygenation, Ginkgo Biloba supports the body's energy production processes. It can provide a natural energy boost, helping individuals stay alert and energized throughout the day.

Antioxidant and Neuroprotective Properties

Ginkgo Biloba is rich in antioxidants, particularly flavonoids and terpenoids. These antioxidants help protect the brain and body from oxidative stress, which is associated with various health conditions, including cognitive decline and aging.

The antioxidant properties of Ginkgo Biloba contribute to its neuroprotective effects. It can help reduce inflammation in the brain, support neuronal health, and promote overall brain function. This makes Ginkgo Biloba a valuable herb for maintaining brain health and potentially slowing down cognitive aging.

How to Incorporate Ginkgo Biloba

Ginkgo Biloba can be consumed in various forms to harness its cognitive-enhancing and energizing benefits:

Supplements: Ginkgo Biloba supplements are widely available in capsule or tablet form. Follow the recommended dosage instructions on the product label.

Tea: Brew Ginkgo Biloba tea using the dried leaves or pre-made tea bags. Enjoy a cup of warm tea to relax and energize.

Tinctures: Ginkgo Biloba tinctures can be added to water or juice for a convenient way to consume the herb.

Extracts: Ginkgo Biloba extracts are often used in natural health products and can be added to beverages or used topically.

It's important to note that while Ginkgo Biloba is generally considered safe, it may interact with certain medications, particularly blood thinners. It is always advisable to consult with a healthcare professional before incorporating Ginkgo Biloba or any herbal supplement into your routine, especially if you have any underlying health conditions.

In conclusion, Ginkgo Biloba is an ancient herb with a long history of traditional use for cognitive enhancement and energy support. Its ability to improve blood flow to the brain, provide antioxidant protection, and enhance cognitive function makes it a valuable addition to a holistic approach to brain health and overall well-being. As with any herbal remedy, moderation and consultation with a healthcare professional are essential for safe and effective use.

21. Schisandra Berry: An Adaptogenic Herb for Energy, Focus, and Resilience

Schisandra Berry, scientifically known as Schisandra chinensis, is an ancient herb that has been used for centuries in traditional Chinese medicine. It is native to East Asia and is renowned for its adaptogenic properties, which help the body adapt to stress and promote overall well-being. Schisandra Berry is often referred to as the "five-flavor fruit" due to its unique combination of sweet, sour, salty, bitter, and pungent flavors.

Energy Boosting and Endurance

Schisandra Berry is known for its energizing effects, making it an excellent choice for individuals seeking a natural boost in energy levels and physical endurance. It contains active compounds called lignans, which are believed to be responsible for its energizing properties.

These lignans work by enhancing mitochondrial function, improving cellular energy production, and increasing overall stamina. Schisandra Berry can help combat fatigue, enhance physical performance, and provide a sustained source of energy throughout the day. Its adaptogenic nature also helps the body adapt to physical stress, making it beneficial for athletes and individuals with active lifestyles.

Focus and Cognitive Enhancement

In addition to its energizing effects, Schisandra Berry is recognized for its positive impact on cognitive function and focus. It has been traditionally used to improve mental clarity, enhance concentration, and support overall brain health.

Research suggests that Schisandra Berry may improve cognitive performance by increasing acetylcholine levels in the brain, a neurotransmitter crucial for memory and learning. It also helps protect brain cells from oxidative stress and supports the growth and repair of neurons. Schisandra Berry's adaptogenic properties contribute to improved focus, mental resilience, and cognitive flexibility.

Stress Relief and Adaptogenic Benefits

One of the key advantages of Schisandra Berry is its adaptogenic properties, which help the body adapt to various forms of stress, both physical and mental. It modulates the stress response by regulating the hypothalamic-pituitary-adrenal (HPA) axis, a key component of the body's stress response system.

By reducing the negative impact of stress on the body, Schisandra Berry promotes a sense of calm and balance. It can help individuals manage stress more effectively, improve mood, and enhance overall resilience. Its adaptogenic nature makes it a valuable herb for individuals facing high-stress situations or seeking to improve their stress management skills.

How to Incorporate Schisandra Berry

Schisandra Berry can be consumed in various forms to harness its energizing, cognitive-enhancing, and adaptogenic benefits:

Supplements: Schisandra Berry supplements are available in capsule or tablet form. Follow the recommended dosage instructions on the product label.

Tea: Brew Schisandra Berry tea using the dried berries or pre-made tea bags. Enjoy a cup of warm tea to relax and energize.

Tinctures: Schisandra Berry tinctures can be added to water or juice for a convenient way to consume the herb.

Powder: Schisandra Berry powder can be mixed into smoothies, yogurt, or oatmeal for a nutritional boost.

It's important to note that while Schisandra Berry is generally considered safe, it may interact with certain medications, particularly those affecting the liver. It is always advisable to consult with a healthcare professional before incorporating Schisandra Berry or any herbal supplement into your routine, especially if you have any underlying health conditions.

In conclusion, Schisandra Berry is an ancient adaptogenic herb with a unique combination of energizing, cognitive-enhancing, and stress-relieving properties. Its ability to boost energy, improve focus, and promote resilience makes it a valuable addition to a holistic approach to health and well-being. As with any herbal remedy, moderation and consultation with a healthcare professional are key to ensuring safe and effective use.

22. Eleuthero (Siberian Ginseng): An Adaptogenic Herb for Energy and Focus

Eleuthero, also known as Siberian Ginseng, is an adaptogenic herb that has been used for centuries in traditional Chinese and Russian medicine. It is native to the forests of Siberia and has gained recognition for its ability to enhance energy levels, improve focus, and support overall well-being.

Energy Boosting Properties

Eleuthero is renowned for its energizing effects, making it a popular choice for individuals seeking a natural boost in energy and stamina. It contains active compounds called eleutherosides, which are believed to be responsible for its energizing properties.

These compounds work by stimulating the body's natural energy production processes and enhancing overall vitality. Eleuthero can help combat fatigue, increase physical endurance, and promote a sense of vigor and mental alertness. Its adaptogenic nature allows it to adapt to the body's needs, providing a balanced and sustainable source of energy.

Focus and Cognitive Enhancement

In addition to its energizing effects, Eleuthero is known for its positive impact on cognitive function and focus. It has been traditionally used to enhance mental clarity, improve concentration, and support overall brain health.

Research suggests that Eleuthero may improve cognitive performance by increasing blood flow to the brain and enhancing oxygen and nutrient delivery to brain cells. It can help improve memory, attention span, and overall mental performance.

Eleuthero's adaptogenic properties also contribute to stress resilience, allowing individuals to maintain focus and concentration even under challenging conditions.

Immune System Support

Eleuthero is not only beneficial for energy and focus but also for supporting the immune system. It has been studied for its immunomodulatory effects, which help regulate and strengthen the body's immune response.

The adaptogenic properties of Eleuthero help the body adapt to various stressors, including physical and mental stress. By modulating the immune system, Eleuthero can enhance its ability to fight off infections, reduce inflammation, and promote overall immune health. This makes it a valuable herb for individuals looking to boost their immune system and maintain overall well-being.

How to Incorporate Eleuthero

Eleuthero can be consumed in various forms to harness its energizing, cognitive-enhancing, and immune-supporting benefits:

Supplements: Eleuthero supplements are widely available in capsule or tablet form. Follow the recommended dosage instructions on the product label.

Tea: Brew Eleuthero tea using the dried root or pre-made tea bags. Enjoy a cup of warm tea to relax and energize.

Tinctures: Eleuthero tinctures can be added to water or juice for a convenient way to consume the herb.

Powder: Eleuthero powder can be mixed into smoothies, yogurt, or oatmeal for a nutritional boost.

It's important to note that while Eleuthero is generally considered safe, it may interact with certain medications, particularly those affecting the immune system. It is always advisable to consult with a healthcare professional before incorporating Eleuthero or any herbal supplement into your routine, especially if you have any underlying health conditions.

In conclusion, Eleuthero is an adaptogenic herb with a wide range of benefits, including enhanced energy levels, improved focus, and immune system support. Its ability to adapt to the body's needs and provide a balanced source of energy makes it a valuable addition to a holistic approach to health and well-being. As with any herbal remedy, moderation and consultation with a healthcare professional are essential for safe and effective use.

23. Green Tea and Coffee: A Dynamic Duo for Cognitive Enhancement

Cognitive Benefits and Focus

Green tea is a popular beverage known for its numerous health benefits, including its positive impact on cognitive function. It contains a unique combination of compounds, such as caffeine, L-theanine, and polyphenols, which work synergistically to enhance focus and mental performance. The caffeine in green tea provides a mild stimulant effect, improving alertness and concentration, while L-theanine promotes relaxation and reduces mental fatigue.

The polyphenols in green tea, particularly catechins, are powerful antioxidants that protect brain cells from oxidative damage. Research suggests that these polyphenols may improve memory, learning abilities, and overall cognitive function. Green tea's ability to enhance focus and protect brain health makes it an excellent choice for cognitive support.

Coffee, another widely consumed beverage, also offers cognitive benefits. It is primarily known for its caffeine content, which acts as a central nervous system stimulant, increasing alertness and improving mental performance. Caffeine in coffee has been shown to enhance focus, attention, and reaction time, making it a popular choice for individuals seeking a mental boost.

In addition to caffeine, coffee contains a variety of polyphenols, including chlorogenic acids, which have antioxidant properties. These polyphenols contribute to coffee's potential brain-health benefits by reducing inflammation and protecting against cognitive decline.

Research on Caffeine and Polyphenols

Numerous studies have explored the impact of caffeine and polyphenols on cognitive function. Research suggests that moderate caffeine intake, as found in green tea and coffee, can improve cognitive performance, particularly in tasks requiring sustained attention and mental effort. Caffeine's ability to enhance focus and alertness makes it a valuable tool for cognitive enhancement.

The polyphenols in green tea and coffee have also been studied for their potential brain-health benefits. These compounds have been linked to improved memory, reduced risk of cognitive decline, and protection against neurodegenerative diseases. The combination of caffeine and polyphenols in these beverages creates a synergistic effect, maximizing their cognitive-enhancing properties.

Guidelines for Consumption

To optimize cognitive support, it is recommended to consume green tea and coffee in moderation. Green tea, with its lower caffeine content, can be enjoyed throughout the day, providing a steady source of focus and relaxation. Coffee, due to its higher caffeine content, is best consumed in the morning or early afternoon to avoid disrupting sleep patterns.

It is important to note that individual tolerance to caffeine varies, and excessive consumption may lead to adverse effects such as jitters, anxiety, or insomnia. It is advisable to monitor your caffeine intake and adjust accordingly to find the right balance for your body.

Potential Side Effects and Considerations

While green tea and coffee offer cognitive benefits, it is essential to be aware of potential side effects and considerations. Excessive caffeine intake can lead to increased heart rate, insomnia, and gastrointestinal discomfort. Individuals with certain medical conditions, such as anxiety disorders or heart problems, should exercise caution and consult with a healthcare professional before increasing their caffeine intake.

Additionally, it is important to choose high-quality, organic green tea and coffee to minimize the risk of exposure to pesticides and other contaminants. Opting for loose-leaf tea and freshly ground coffee beans can ensure a more controlled and healthier experience.

In conclusion, green tea and coffee, when consumed in moderation, can provide a dynamic duo for cognitive enhancement. Their unique combination of caffeine, L-theanine, and polyphenols offers a range of benefits, including improved focus, mental performance, and brain health. As with any dietary choice, it is crucial to listen to your body and make informed decisions based on your individual needs and preferences.

24. Energy Drinks: A Controversial Topic for Focus and Health

Energy drinks have become increasingly popular, especially among young adults and individuals seeking a quick boost in energy and focus. These beverages are marketed as powerful stimulants, often containing a unique blend of ingredients designed to enhance mental and physical performance. However, the question of whether energy drinks are good or bad for focus and overall health remains a topic of debate and concern.

Energy drinks typically contain a combination of stimulants, including caffeine, taurine, and various B-vitamins. Let's explore the key ingredients and their potential impact on focus and health:

Caffeine

Caffeine is the primary stimulant in energy drinks, known for its ability to increase alertness, improve focus, and enhance physical performance. It works by blocking adenosine receptors in the brain, leading to increased dopamine and norepinephrine levels, which promote wakefulness and cognitive function.

While moderate caffeine intake can provide benefits, excessive consumption can lead to adverse effects such as jitters, anxiety, insomnia, and increased heart rate. The high caffeine content in energy drinks, often exceeding the recommended daily limit, raises concerns about potential health risks.

Taurine

Taurine is an amino acid naturally found in the body and is commonly added to energy drinks. It is believed to enhance physical performance and improve cognitive function. Taurine has been studied for its potential antioxidant and anti-inflammatory properties, which may contribute to overall health.

However, the exact mechanism of action and long-term effects of taurine in energy drinks are not fully understood. More research is needed to determine its safety and efficacy when consumed in high doses.

B-Vitamins

Energy drinks often contain high doses of B-vitamins, particularly B6, B12, and niacin. These vitamins play crucial roles in energy metabolism and brain function. While B-vitamins are essential for overall health, excessive intake can lead to adverse effects, including skin flushing, nausea, and nerve damage.

Impact on Focus and Health

The effects of energy drinks on focus and cognitive function are complex and vary among individuals. While the stimulants in energy drinks can provide a temporary boost in alertness and focus, their long-term impact on cognitive performance is not well established.

Research suggests that excessive consumption of energy drinks may lead to negative health outcomes. The high caffeine content can cause dehydration, increased blood pressure, and cardiovascular strain. Additionally, the combination of stimulants and sugar in energy drinks may contribute to weight gain, dental issues, and an increased risk of type 2 diabetes.

Guidelines and Considerations

If you choose to consume energy drinks, it is essential to do so in moderation and with caution. Here are some guidelines and considerations:

Limit your intake to occasional use, especially during periods of high mental or physical demand.

Choose energy drinks with lower caffeine content and avoid excessive consumption.

Be mindful of the sugar content and opt for sugar-free or low-sugar options to minimize the risk of weight gain and dental problems.

Consider alternative sources of energy and focus, such as a balanced diet, regular exercise, and adequate sleep.

Consult with a healthcare professional, especially if you have underlying health conditions or are taking medications, to ensure safe consumption.

Energy drinks can provide a temporary boost in energy and focus, but their long-term effects on health and cognitive function are not fully understood. While the ingredients in energy drinks may offer some benefits, excessive consumption can lead to adverse health outcomes. It is crucial to approach energy drinks with caution and prioritize overall health and well-being through a balanced lifestyle.

25. Embracing a Low-Sugar Lifestyle: A Path to Enhanced Focus, Weight Loss, and Overall Well-being

Ditching Sugar for Focus and Gut Health

Reducing sugar intake, especially from sources like high-fructose corn syrup (HFCS) in soft drinks, can have a profound impact on various aspects of health, including focus, gut health, and overall well-being. Here's how embracing a low-sugar lifestyle can benefit you:

Boosting Focus

Excessive sugar consumption, particularly from refined sugars and HFCS, can lead to blood sugar spikes and crashes, affecting focus and mental clarity. By reducing sugar intake, you stabilize blood sugar levels, providing a consistent source of energy for the brain. This stability enhances focus, concentration, and cognitive performance, allowing you to stay mentally sharp throughout the day.

Supporting Gut Health and Candida

The gut microbiome plays a crucial role in overall health, including brain function. A diet high in sugar, especially refined sugars and HFCS, can disrupt the balance of gut bacteria, promoting the overgrowth of harmful bacteria like Candida. Candida overgrowth can lead to various health issues, including brain fog, fatigue, and digestive problems.

By eliminating or significantly reducing sugar intake, you create an environment in your gut that favors the growth of beneficial bacteria. This supports a healthy gut microbiome, which, in turn, positively impacts brain health and cognitive function. A balanced gut microbiome can enhance focus, improve mood, and reduce inflammation, contributing to overall well-being.

Aiding Weight Loss and Slowing Aging

Reducing sugar intake is a powerful strategy for weight loss and promoting healthy aging. Here's how:

Sugar, especially in the form of added sugars and HFCS, is highly caloric and can contribute to weight gain. By cutting back on sugar, you reduce your overall calorie intake, making it easier to create a calorie deficit and promote weight loss. Additionally, stabilizing blood sugar levels through a low-sugar diet can help reduce cravings and promote a healthier relationship with food.

Slowing Aging

Excessive sugar consumption has been linked to accelerated aging and an increased risk of age-related diseases. Sugar can lead to a process called glycation, where sugar molecules attach to proteins, causing damage and inflammation. This process contributes to the development of chronic conditions such as diabetes, cardiovascular disease, and cognitive decline.

By reducing sugar intake, you minimize the risk of glycation and its associated health issues. A low-sugar diet can help preserve collagen and elastin in the skin, promoting a more youthful appearance. Additionally, the anti-inflammatory effects of a low-sugar diet can support overall health and potentially slow down the aging process.

Practical Tips for a Low-Sugar Lifestyle

Here are some practical tips to help you embrace a low-sugar lifestyle:

Read food labels carefully and choose products with minimal added sugars.

Opt for natural sweeteners like stevia or erythritol in moderation.

Satisfy your sweet tooth with whole foods like fruits, which provide natural sugars along with essential nutrients.

Gradually reduce your sugar intake to allow your taste buds to adjust.

Stay hydrated with water or herbal teas instead of sugary drinks.

Experiment with sugar-free alternatives and recipes to enjoy your favorite treats without the sugar overload.

Seek support from friends, family, or support groups to stay motivated and accountable.

Remember, a low-sugar lifestyle is not about deprivation but rather about making conscious choices to support your health and well-being. By reducing sugar intake, you can boost your focus, support gut health, aid weight loss, and potentially slow down the aging process. You are also lowering your risk for cancer by reducing sugar intake with some recommendations at consuming 5 or less grams of sugar per day. (Thats about one teaspoon.)

26. Foods for Focus: Nourishing Your Brain for Optimal Cognitive Function

Maintaining optimal cognitive function and focus is essential for overall well-being and productivity. The foods we consume play a crucial role in supporting brain health and enhancing our mental performance. By incorporating nutrient-rich foods into our diet, we can provide our brains with the necessary fuel to stay sharp, focused, and energized.

Brain-Boosting Nutrients and Their Sources

Several key nutrients have been identified as essential for cognitive function and brain health. Here are some of the most beneficial nutrients and their natural sources:

Omega-3 Fatty Acids

Omega-3 fatty acids, particularly docosahexaenoic acid (DHA) and eicosapentaenoic acid (EPA), are crucial for brain health. These healthy fats support cognitive function, improve memory, and reduce inflammation.

Sources: Fatty fish like salmon, mackerel, and sardines are excellent sources of omega-3s. Walnuts, flaxseeds, chia seeds, and hemp seeds also contain omega-3 fatty acids.

B-Vitamins

B-vitamins, including B6, B12, and folate, play a vital role in brain function and the production of neurotransmitters. They support cognitive performance, mood regulation, and overall brain health.

Sources: Animal-based foods such as meat, fish, eggs, and dairy products are rich in B-vitamins. Plant-based sources include legumes, whole grains, nuts, and seeds.

Antioxidants

Antioxidants help protect brain cells from oxidative damage caused by free radicals. They reduce inflammation and support overall brain health.

Sources: Berries (blueberries, strawberries, raspberries), dark chocolate, green tea, spinach, and broccoli are excellent sources of antioxidants.

Choline

Choline is an essential nutrient for brain development and function. It supports the production of acetylcholine, a neurotransmitter involved in memory and cognitive processes.

Sources: Eggs, liver, fish, soybeans, and broccoli are good sources of choline.

Magnesium

Magnesium is crucial for brain health and cognitive function. It plays a role in neurotransmitter release and helps regulate brain activity.

Sources: Leafy green vegetables like spinach and kale, nuts, seeds, whole grains, and avocados are rich in magnesium.

Superfoods for Energy and Focus: A Comprehensive Guide

Fruits for Energy and Cognitive Enhancement

Berries: Nature's Brain Boosters

Berries, including blueberries, strawberries, raspberries, and blackberries, are true superfoods for cognitive health. They are packed with antioxidants, particularly flavonoids, which have been linked to improved memory, enhanced focus, and reduced mental fatigue. The antioxidants in berries protect brain cells from oxidative stress, promoting overall brain function and longevity.

Citrus Fruits: Vitamin C Powerhouses

Citrus fruits, such as oranges, lemons, limes, and grapefruits, are renowned for their high vitamin C content. Vitamin C is a powerful antioxidant that plays a crucial role in maintaining cognitive function and supporting the immune system. It helps reduce inflammation in the brain, improves blood flow, and enhances overall cognitive performance.

Avocados: Healthy Fats for Brain Health

Avocados are unique fruits that offer a rich source of monounsaturated fats, which are essential for brain health and cognitive function. These healthy fats provide a steady release of energy, keeping your brain fueled throughout the day. Avocados are also packed with vitamin E, an antioxidant that protects brain cells from damage and supports overall brain health.

Tropical Fruits: Energy-Boosting Delights

Tropical fruits like mangoes, pineapples, and papayas are not only delicious but also packed with nutrients that support energy and focus. Mangoes are rich in vitamin C and fiber, promoting stable energy levels and digestive health. Pineapples contain bromelain, an enzyme with anti-inflammatory properties, which can enhance cognitive function. Papayas are a good source of vitamin A, supporting eye health and overall brain function.

Vegetables: Nutrient-Dense Brain Fuel

Leafy Greens: Nutritional Powerhouses

Leafy green vegetables, such as spinach, kale, Swiss chard, and collard greens, are true nutritional powerhouses. They are packed with vitamins, minerals, and antioxidants, making them essential for brain health and cognitive function. Leafy greens are rich in folate, a B-vitamin that plays a vital role in brain development, memory, and cognitive performance.

Broccoli: A Cruciferous Brain Booster

Broccoli is a cruciferous vegetable that offers a wide range of benefits for brain health. It is an excellent source of vitamin K, which is essential for cognitive function and brain development. Vitamin K helps improve memory, focus, and overall brain performance. Broccoli also contains sulforaphane, a compound with potent antioxidant and anti-inflammatory properties, protecting brain cells from damage.

Sweet Potatoes: Complex Carbohydrate Power

Sweet potatoes are a fantastic source of complex carbohydrates, providing a steady release of energy and sustaining focus throughout the day. They are rich in vitamin A, which is crucial for brain development, vision, and immune function. Sweet potatoes also contain antioxidants like beta-carotene, protecting brain cells from oxidative stress.

Bell Peppers: Colorful Brain Nutrition

Bell peppers, available in various colors like red, yellow, and green, are packed with nutrients that support brain health. They are an excellent source of vitamin C, an antioxidant that protects brain cells and enhances cognitive function. Bell peppers also contain vitamin B6, which plays a role in neurotransmitter production, supporting mood and cognitive performance.

Nuts and Seeds: Energy-Dense Brain Snacks

Walnuts: Omega-3 Powerhouses

Walnuts are an exceptional source of omega-3 fatty acids, which are essential for brain health and cognitive function. Omega-3s support brain development, improve memory, and enhance overall cognitive performance. Walnuts are also rich in antioxidants and vitamins, making them a nutritious and energy-dense snack.

Almonds: Healthy Fats and Protein

Almonds are a popular choice for a reason - they offer a perfect balance of healthy fats, protein, and fiber. This combination provides a sustained release of energy, keeping you focused and energized throughout the day. Almonds are also a good source of vitamin E, an antioxidant that protects brain cells and supports cognitive function.

Pumpkin Seeds: Magnesium-Rich Superfood

Pumpkin seeds are a nutritional powerhouse, packed with magnesium, zinc, and healthy fats. Magnesium is essential for brain function, mood regulation, and cognitive performance. Zinc plays a crucial role in brain development and memory. Pumpkin seeds also provide a good amount of protein, supporting overall energy levels and muscle health.

Chia Seeds: Tiny Superfood for Energy

Chia seeds are tiny but mighty seeds that offer a range of benefits for energy and focus. They are an excellent source of omega-3 fatty acids, fiber, and protein. Chia seeds provide a sustained release of energy, keeping you energized and focused for longer periods. They are also rich in antioxidants, supporting overall brain health.

Additional Superfoods for Energy and Focus

Dark Chocolate: Brain-Boosting Indulgence

Dark chocolate, with a high cocoa content, is a delicious superfood for brain health. It contains flavonoids, which have antioxidant and anti-inflammatory properties, supporting cognitive function and blood flow to the brain. Dark chocolate also contains caffeine and theobromine, providing a gentle energy boost without the jitters.

Seaweed: Nutrient-Rich Ocean Superfood

Seaweed, including varieties like nori, wakame, and kombu, is a nutrient-dense superfood. It is rich in iodine, which is essential for thyroid function and overall brain health. Seaweed also contains vitamins, minerals, and antioxidants, supporting cognitive function and overall well-being.

Tips for Incorporating Energy-Boosting Superfoods

Start your day with a nutritious breakfast that includes a variety of fruits, vegetables, and nuts.

Aim for a colorful plate by incorporating different colored fruits and vegetables, each offering unique nutrients.

Snack on nuts, seeds, and dried fruits throughout the day to maintain energy levels and focus.

Add berries to your morning smoothie, yogurt, or oatmeal for an antioxidant-rich boost.

Incorporate leafy greens into salads, soups, or stir-fries for a nutrient-dense meal.

Choose whole grain carbohydrates like quinoa, brown rice, or whole wheat bread for sustained energy release.

Stay hydrated by drinking plenty of water and herbal teas, such as green tea or chamomile.

Limit your intake of processed foods, sugary snacks, and excessive caffeine, as they can lead to energy crashes and decreased focus.

Experiment with different superfoods and recipes to find what works best for your taste preferences and energy needs.

Remember, a well-balanced diet that includes a variety of superfoods can provide the necessary nutrients to support optimal energy levels, enhance focus, and promote overall brain health. By incorporating these foods into your daily routine, you can fuel your body and mind for peak performance and well-being.